AROMATHERAPY
FOR ALL

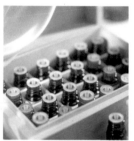 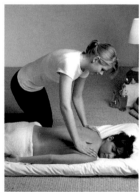 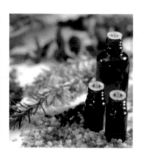

JOANNA TREVELYAN

Haldane Mason

First published in the UK in 2001 by
Haldane Mason Ltd
59 Chepstow Road
London W2 5BP
email: haldane.mason@dial.pipex.com

ISBN: 1-902463-47-1

A HALDANE MASON BOOK

Editor: Ambreen Husain
Designer: Rachel Clark
Models: Asa Lundqvist Dip.LCM, Cristiane Guida de Camargo

Colour reproduction by CK Litho Ltd, UK
Printed in China

Picture Acknowledgements
All photographs by Sue Ford, with the exception of the following:
Sydney Francis 5; Werner Forman Archive 4, 9.

The author and publishers would like to thank Fresh & Wild in Notting Hill, London,
for supplying the essential oils box used on page 29.

Important
The information in this book is generally applicable but is not tailored to specific
circumstances or individuals. The author and publishers can accept no responsibility for any
problems arising from following the information given in this book. Safety information is
supplied which should be read before attempting to give an aromatherapy massage. Any of
the oils can produce an allergic reaction. If in doubt about any of the techniques described,
please consult your doctor or aromatherapy practitioner.

Contents

Introduction

Whose spirits have not been lifted by the smell of fresh parsley in a salad, or the heady scent of jasmine on a summer evening? We seem to know instinctively that the marvellous aromas of herbs and flowers are good for us. Since earliest times we have included them in our beauty preparations, medicines, cuisine and religions. It is from this intuitive understanding that modern aromatherapy has developed.

Aromatherapy can be seen as a modern interpretation of ancient knowledge. Archaeologists have found evidence that the people of the Indus Valley (in present-day Pakistan) knew how to distil oils as far back as 3000 BC. In fact, many ancient cultures made use of aromatics: Chinese and Indian writings dating from 2000 BC describe the use of aromatics for medicinal and religious practices; the Ancient Egyptians had been using them since 3000 BC for

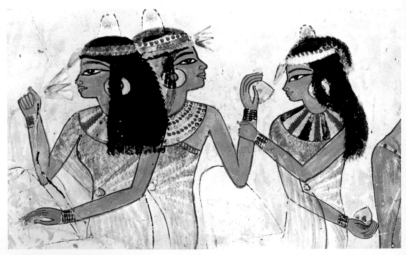

In Ancient Egypt, ladies at a feast would wear perfumed ointment cones. These would slowly melt over the course of the evening, scenting their hair and necks.

perfumes, in embalming practices and in their medicines; and the Ancient Greeks added to Egyptian practices – for example, by using olive oil to absorb plant aromas.

As the Romans employed Greek physicians, the use of aromatics spread throughout the Roman Empire. The Arabs in turn made translations of the Graeco-Roman medical texts and proceeded to take the medicinal use of aromatics to new heights. One of the most famous Arab doctors was Abu Ali Ibn Sina, or Avicenna as he became known in the West (AD 980–1037). As well as describing some 800 plants and their effects on the body, he also developed a method of distilling essential oils.

In Europe, the use of herbs and other plants dates back to earliest times. By the Middle Ages aromatic oils from the East were brought to Europe by traders and by the Crusaders (who returned from their Holy Wars with the knowledge of how to distil them). During the Renaissance the distillation process was industrialized, and chemists began to investigate the constituents of the oils.

It was a French chemist called René-Maurice Gattefosse who, in 1928, first coined the term aromatherapy. His family owned a perfume factory and, while working

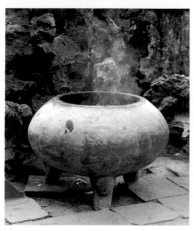

In China, incense burners such as this one are still used at temples.

in his laboratory, Gattefosse burnt his hand. Desperate to relieve the pain, he plunged his hand into a nearby container of neat lavender oil. To his surprise the burns healed within hours, leaving no scars. This prompted him to explore the properties of other oils. In his writings on the subject he always referred to 'aromatherapie' and the term stuck.

In the 1950s another Frenchman, Dr Jean Valnet, began using essential oils in his medical practice. His success inspired others to follow his lead, and stimulated research. In other countries the popularity of aromatherapy is more recent, and in some it is still thought of as a beauty treatment rather than as a therapy.

What
is
Aromatherapy?

Aromatherapy has different meanings
for different people: a beauty treatment,
a kind of massage therapy that smells good,
or an effective treatment for all sorts of health
problems. Each is in common parlance today.
The word 'aromatherapy' simply means
'treatment with the use of fragrance' (although
the word aroma actually comes from the Greek
for spice), so we must look elsewhere for a
clearer definition.

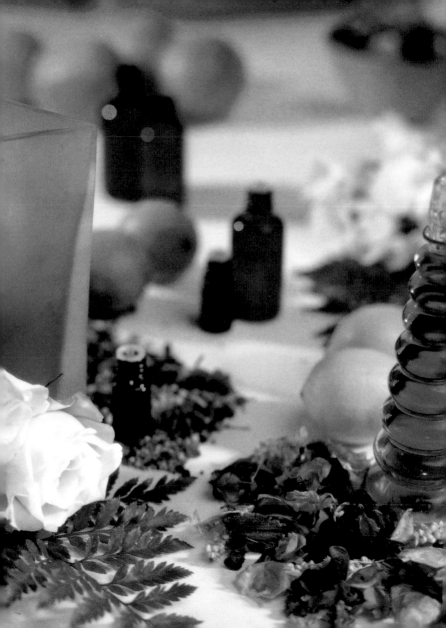

A natural therapy

Aromatherapy uses essential oils extracted from herbs, flowers, fruits and trees. These oils give the plant its 'aroma'. They also contain complex chemical compounds, many of which have been found to have psychological or physiological effects. The basis of aromatherapy is that, when massaged into the skin, inhaled or, in some cases, consumed, essential oils interact with our bodies, and can therefore be used to enhance our sense of well-being, alleviate stress and help with a variety of health problems.

Research into aromatherapy

While aromatherapy is without doubt extremely popular, there has not been much research to support many of its therapeutic claims. At a very basic level there is evidence that suggests 'aromas' have a psychological effect; and research on how essential oils may affect the nervous system has found that changes in electrical activity of the brain (stimulation or sedation) often correlate with the traditional properties ascribed to particular essential oils. However, it is also known that these changes may be the result of our expectations rather than an inherent effect of the aroma.

Although many oils have recognized theraputic properties, relatively few clinical trials of essential oils have been done. Trials that have been done suggest that:

• peppermint oil is of benefit for irritable bowel syndrome

• tea tree oil has anti-fungal and anti-bacterial properties, and is an effective treatment for certain skin infections and also for MRSA (a bug that is resistant to many other treatments)

• lavender oil will heal burns and cold sores, and helps relieve stress and insomnia

• rosemary and Spanish oregano can be used to treat bacterial infections

• thyme oil is good for migraine

• many essential oils ease breathing in respiratory tract infections when inhaled or used in massage.

Also, an unpublished, but extensive, trial by the International Federation of Aromatherapists suggests aromatherapy is an effective treatment for endometriosis (inflammation of the mucus membrane that lines the uterus).

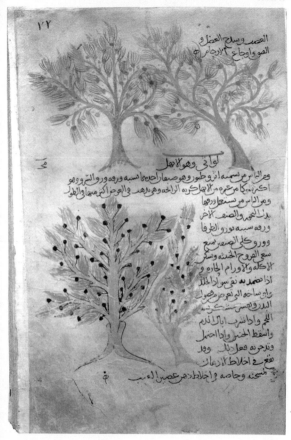

The Arabs translated the writings of Dioscorides, an Ancient Greek scholar who wrote in detail about the medicinal properties of plants. Arab doctors went on to develop the medicinal use of aromatics even further.

Research has shown that essential oils:
- often have antiseptic qualities, and show anti-microbial activity
- can increase the sedative effect of massage
- show anti-inflammatory, digestive, sedative and pain-relieving properties
- can be absorbed into the bloodstream by inhalation and topical application.

Aromatherapy in health care

Aromatherapy is being used by doctors and nurses in many hospitals and surgeries around the world. Patients have certainly benefited from this, reporting improvements in their health and well-being. Here are just a few examples of its use.

- Inhaled lavender oil is regularly used with older patients in long-stay hospital wards to help with sleep problems. Interestingly, the oil not only helps patients sleep, but also improves daytime wakefulness and alertness.

- In Intensive Care wards, foot massage with neroli or lavender oil has helped reduce anxiety among patients who have had heart surgery.

- Aromatherapy massage with essential oils is helping epilepsy patients reduce the frequency with which they experience seizures. Patients choose from a range of essential oils said to be either arousing or calming.

- Midwives have found that massage with clary sage oil is effective in reducing anxiety, fear and pain during labour.

- Massage with essential oils is regularly used as a relaxing treatment for cancer patients.

- Tea tree oil has been used as an anti-fungal treatment for candida and stomatitis (inflammation of the mucus membrane of the mouth) among patients in a hospice setting.

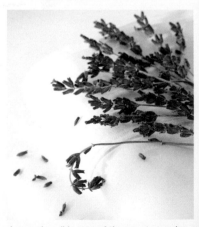

Lavender oil is one of the most popular essential oils among health professionals.

Safety with essential oils

Although most essential oils are perfectly safe for home use, they are highly concentrated and need to be used with care. The guidelines given here highlight potential hazards and how to avoid them.

Using essential oils safely

There are some basic safety guidelines which you should follow when using essential oils. The key points are:

- always store essential oils out of reach of children and pets
- keep essential oils away from naked flames as they are flammable
- never take essential oils internally
- unless otherwise stated, essential oils should always be diluted before use
- wash your hands with undiluted washing-up liquid if you get essential oils on them
- avoid rubbing your eyes when working with essential oils, and if you do get oils in them, rinse immediately with warm water
- to avoid irritation to the skin or an allergic reaction, do a patch test (see below for details) before trying a new essential oil on yourself or anyone else
- avoid the prolonged use of the same essential oil, and regularly take a break from using essential oils generally as, over time, skin can become sensitive from both actual and airborne contact.

Doing a patch test

Before using any new essential oil it is worth testing a drop of diluted essential oil (see Aromatherapy at Home for guidelines on dilution) on the inside of your wrist or elbow. Cover the area with a plaster and leave for about 12 hours. If after this time there is any redness or itching, do not use that essential oil. If you do have an adverse reaction, you can put a little almond oil on the area, and then wash with cold water. If the reaction persists, consult your doctor.

When essential oils should not be used

People differ in opinion on when essential oils can and cannot be used, but the best advice has to be to err on the side of caution. Here is a list of situations when essential oils either should not be used or should be used with care.

- During pregnancy – consult an obstetrician and a qualified aromatherapist about which oils are safe, and only use oils well diluted.

- People with epilepsy – they can be adversely affected by certain essential oils, so discuss the use of any oils with their consultant and a qualified aromatherapist.

- People suffering from asthma – they should check essential oils with their doctor and a qualified aromatherapist before use. Any essential oils used should be well diluted.

- People taking medication or homeopathic remedies – check with their doctor or homeopath before using essential oils.

- Babies and young children – they have delicate skin and essential oils should be used on them only when extremely well diluted.

- People with sensitive skin – use essential oils with care and well diluted.

- People with skin allergies – take professional advice before trying aromatherapy.

- Citrus oils seem to increase our sensitivity to the sun, so avoid exposure to the sun or a sunbed for at least six hours after use.

- Essential oils that are said to be relaxing can cause drowsiness and should not be used if you are going to drive or use machinery shortly afterwards.

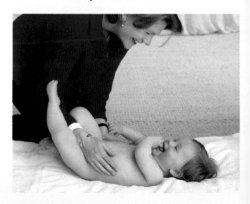

Potentially hazardous essential oils

There are some essential oils which are potentially very toxic, but they are not easily available. Some of those listed here as hazardous are used in perfumes, food flavourings, medicines and medicinal products and, on occasion, by experienced aromatherapists. They are not, however, recommended for home use. For the amateur, it is wise to keep to the essential oils described in the next section.

Common Name	Latin Name	Common Name	Latin Name
Arnica	*Arnica montana*	Narcissus	*Narcissus poeticus*
Bitter Almond	*Prunus dulcis var. amara*	Mountain (dwarf) pine	*Pinus mugo (P. pumilio)*
Boldo leaf	*Peumus boldus*	Pennyroyal	*Mentha pulegium*
Broom	*Cytisus scoparius*	Rue	*Ruta graveolens*
Buchu	*Barosma betulina*	Sassafras	*Sassafras varifolium*
Calamus	*Acorus calamus*	Savine	*Juniperus sabina*
Cinnamon bark	*Cinnamomum cassia*	Tansy	*Tanacetum vulgare*
Camphor (brown, yellow, and white)	*Cinnamomum camphora*	Thuja	*Thuja occidentali*
Chervil	*Anthriscus cerefolium*	Tonka	*Diperyx odorata oppositiflora*
Horseradish	*Cochlearia armoracia*	Wintergreen	*Gaultheria procumbens*
Jaborandi	*Pilocarpus microphyllus*	Wormwood	*Artemisia absinthium*
Mugwort	*Artemisia vulgaris*	Wormseed	*Chenopodium ambrosioides*

It is the essential oil from these plants that is potentially dangerous, not necessarily the plant it is extracted from. The plant may well be commonly and safely used in cooking, herbal medicine or homeopathic remedies.

A-Z
of
Essential
Oils

With such a huge choice of essential oils available, it can be difficult to know which ones to purchase. This section describes some commonly used oils including their therapeutic properties, home uses and potential dangers.

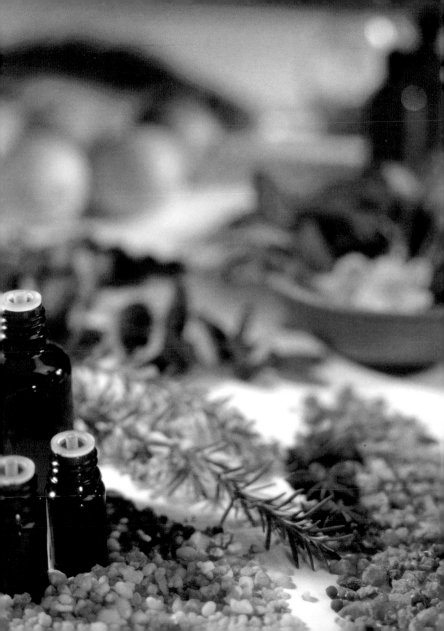

A–Z of essential oils

What are essential oils?

Essential oils are concentrated essences extracted from flowers, leaves, seeds, roots, bark, wood, fruit, spices and herbs. Extraction is generally by steam distillation – a process whereby a specific part of a plant is heated with steam or water, which drives off a mixture of volatile natural chemicals, the essential oil. Other methods used are solvent extraction, a phytonic process using environmentally friendly solvents, super-critical carbon-dioxide extraction, expression or enfleurage.

How do essential oils work?

Essential oils can be absorbed through the skin in small amounts, but when massaged over time most of the molecules of 'aroma' disperse in the air and affect us through smell, and thereby the limbic system (nerve pathways in the brain). Each essential oil is composed of many different chemical components with individual properties. Some components of particular essential oils are absorbed by inhalation, and studies suggest absorption through the skin can occur when inhalation is prevented. However, there is no proof that all, or any, components of essential oils will travel to a given organ and cause a specific effect.

Essential oils are usually categorized as stimulating, relaxing, uplifting and calming, and most have anti-bacterial and antiseptic properties. Some are also anti-viral.

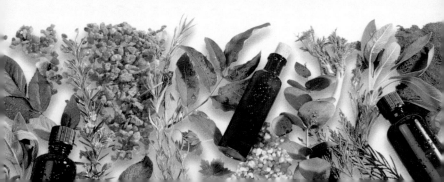

Getting to know essential oils

It would be best to get used to a few oils at first and understand their effects. This list of some commonly used essential oils should give you a good starting point. The actions and uses described here are those ascribed by most aromatherapists.

Allspice *Pimenta dioica*
Scent: Sweet, spicy.
Properties: Stimulant, pain-reliever, antiseptic, digestive aid, muscle relaxant, tonic.
Uses: Poor circulation, muscle and joint problems, chills, congested coughs, bronchitis, digestive problems, depression, nervous exhaustion, neuralgia, stress.
Cautions: Skin irritation and irritation of the mucous membranes. Use well diluted.

Basil, Sweet *Ocimum basilicum*
Scent: Fresh, sweet, spicy, balsamic.
Properties: Stimulant, anti-depressant, antiseptic, tonic, digestive aid.
Uses: Anxiety, negative emotions, depression, mental fatigue, poor memory, catarrh, appetite stimulant, insomnia.
Cautions: Skin irritant, avoid during pregnancy.

Bergamot *Citrus bergamia*
Scent: Fresh, lively, citrus.
Properties: Relaxant, anti-depressant, antiseptic, refreshing.
Uses: Improving moods, depression, anxiety, grief, loss of appetite, oily skin, acne, urinary problems.
Cautions: Skin irritation and photosensitization. Use only well diluted.

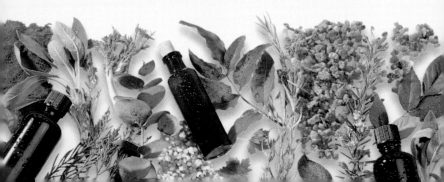

Bois de Rose (Rosewood)
Aniba rosaeodora
Scent: Lightly rosy, woody, spicy.
Properties: Relaxant, calming agent, antiseptic, mild pain-reliever, anti-depressant, tonic, anti-bacterial, aphrodisiac, deodorant, stimulant (for the immune system).
Uses: Skin care, dermatitis, acne, colds, coughs, fever, infections, promoting sleep, calming nerves, mood uplifting.
Cautions: None.

Camomile, Blue (German)
Matricaria recutita
Scent: Pungent, herbaceous, fruity.
Properties: Calming agent, anti-inflammatory, anti-bacterial, antispasmodic.
Uses: Wounds, skin problems, muscle stiffness, joint pain, bronchitis, lung problems, nervous tension, stress, menstrual problems, digestive problems, hay fever and allergies.
Cautions: Occasional skin irritation, avoid during pregnancy.

Camomile, Roman
Chamaemelum nobile
Scent: Pungent, fruity, herbaceous.
Properties: Calming agent, anti-bacterial, relaxant, sedative, anti-inflammatory.
Uses: Insomnia, stress, tension headaches, and same as Blue Camomile.
Cautions: Can cause skin irritation, avoid during pregnancy.

Cedarwood *Cedrus atlantica*
Scent: Fresh, woody.
Properties: Relaxant, sedative, antiseptic, astringent, insecticidal, anti-catarrhal.
Uses: Skin problems, muscle stiffness, joint pain, bronchitis, lung problems, urinary tract problems,

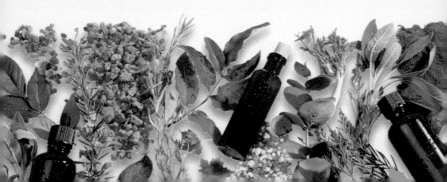

mental exhaustion.
Cautions: Skin irritation and sensitization, use well diluted, avoid during pregnancy.

Clary Sage *Salvia sclarea*
Scent: Herbaceous, hay-like, warm, musky.
Properties: Relaxant, sedative, anti-depressant, aphrodisiac, antiseptic, astringent.
Uses: Depression, panic, shock, anxiety, skin disorders, menstrual and menopausal problems, stress, muscular tension.
Cautions: Large amounts can cause drowsiness, avoid in pregnancy.

Cypress *Cupressus sempervirens*
Scent: Refreshing, piney, lightly spicy and woody.
Properties: Relaxant, astringent, refreshing, anti-cough, antispasmodic.

Uses: Flu, calming irritability and impatience, menstrual and menopausal problems, skin tonic for oily skin, acne, spasmodic coughs.
Cautions: None.

Eucalyptus *Eucalyptus globulus*
Scent: Powerful, camphor-like, sweet, woody.
Properties: Stimulant, uplifting, antiseptic, antispasmodic, expectorant, pain-reliever, anti-viral, anti-bacterial.
Uses: Respiratory tract problems, nasal congestion, chest infections, muscular aches and joint pain, colds, flu, urinary tract infections, mood uplifting, lethargy, insect repellent.
Cautions: Avoid in massage, toxic if consumed, avoid in early pregnancy.

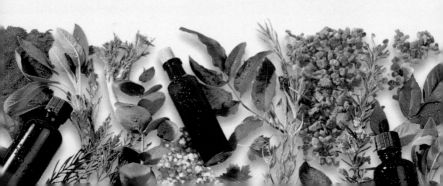

Fennel *Foeniculum vulgare*
Scent: Sweet, delicate, aniseed-like.
Properties: Stimulant, antiseptic, anti-nausea, antispasmodic, anti-fungal.
Uses: Stomach upsets, indigestion, colic, spasmodic coughs, menstrual problems, moodiness, fear, worry.
Cautions: Skin sensitivity, avoid in massage, use low dilution and in moderation. Avoid in pregnancy, with children, with epilepsy.

Frankincense (Olibanum)
Boswellia thurifera
Scent: Warm, spicy, slightly peppery.
Properties: Relaxant, sedative, antiseptic, pain-relieving, astringent, general tonic, comforting.
Uses: Skin care, menstrual problems, asthma, coughs, colds, worry, fear, confusion.
Cautions: Avoid in early pregnancy.

Geranium *Pelargonium graveolens,*
P. odorantissimum **and others**
Scent: Sweet, floral.
Properties: Relaxant, sedative, anti-depressant, antiseptic, astringent, tonic, circulatory, stimulant.
Uses: Balancing hormones, menstrual and menopausal problems, nervous tension, skin problems, herpes, relaxation, mood uplifting, for confidence and self-esteem.
Cautions: Skin irritation.

Jasmine *Jasminum grandiflorum*
Scent: Rich, floral, heady, sweet.
Properties: Relaxant, sedative, anti-depressant, antispasmodic, antiseptic.
Uses: Menstrual problems, impotence, depression, lethargy, mood uplifting, skin problems, in labour.
Cautions: Skin irritation, use well diluted, avoid in pregnancy.

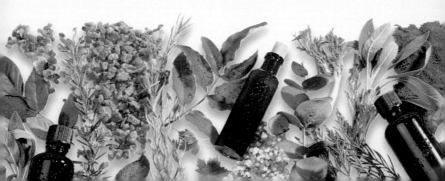

Lavender *Lavandula angustifolia*
or *L. officinalis*
Scent: Floral, sweet, herbaceous.
Properties: Relaxant, sedative,
anti-depressant, antispasmodic,
antiseptic, pain-relieving, anti-nausea.
Uses: There is little this oil cannot be
used for, but especially relaxation,
skin problems, burns, colds, catarrh,
menstrual problems, headaches.
Cautions: Occasionally skin irritation,
avoid in early pregnancy.

Lemon *Citrus limonum*
Scent: Fresh, citrus.
Properties: Stimulating, antiseptic,
astringent, tonic, expectorant,
cleansing.
Uses: Respiratory problems, muscular
aches, arthritis, joint pain, bruises,
flu, colds, warts, verrucas, skin care,
anxiety.
Cautions: Skin irritation, phototoxic,
avoid in steam inhalation.

Marjoram, Sweet
Origanum majorana
Scent: Sweet, warm, camphor-like.
Properties: Calming, sedative,
anti-bacterial, pain-relieving,
antispasmodic, tissue-warming.
Uses: Muscular problems, arthritis,
rheumatism, headaches, migraine,
digestive problems, insomnia, nasal
and sinus congestion, anxiety, grief,
depression.
Cautions: Has a stupefying effect in
excess, avoid during pregnancy.

Myrrh *Commiphora myrrha*
Scent: Spicy, rich, sweet, woody.
Properties: Uplifting, anti-
inflammatory, anti-viral, anti-
bacterial, antispasmodic, healing.
Uses: Skin problems, throat and
chest infections, gingivitis, mouth
ulcers, emotional problems,
depression.
Cautions: Avoid during pregnancy.

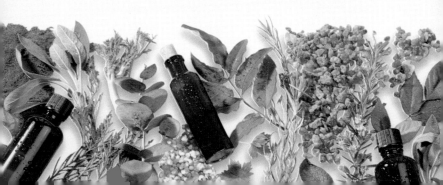

Neroli (Orange blossom)
Citrus aurantium
Scent: Sweet, rich, floral.
Properties: Calming, uplifting, anti-depressant, aphrodisiac, antiseptic, antispasmodic.
Uses: Stress, insomnia, skin problems, balancing moods, nervous tension, menstrual and menopausal problems, phobias.
Cautions: Avoid in early pregnancy.

Orange, Sweet (from rind of fruit)
Citrus sinensis
Scent: Fresh, dry, citrus.
Properties: Stimulant, uplifting, antiseptic, astringent, tonic, antispasmodic.
Uses: Skin care, colds, flu, bronchial congestion, fluid retention, constipation, menstrual and menopausal problems, anxiety, depression.

Cautions: May irritate sensitive skin, possibly phototoxic.

Palmarosa **Cymbopogon martinii**
Scent: Sweet, floral, rosy-geranium.
Properties: Relaxant, antiseptic, tonic, anti-bacterial, digestive.
Uses: Skin infections, anorexia, digestive problems, stress, nervous exhaustion.
Cautions: None.

Patchouli **Pogostemon cablin**
Scent: Balsamic, sweet woody, musky.
Properties: Stimulant, uplifting, stomach calming, anti-inflammatory, anti-depressant, anti-bacterial, anti-viral, tonic, antiseptic, astringent, aphrodisiac.
Uses: Skin care, skin problems, depression, lethargy, scalp problems, oily hair, fungal infections, stress.
Cautions: Can cause headaches.

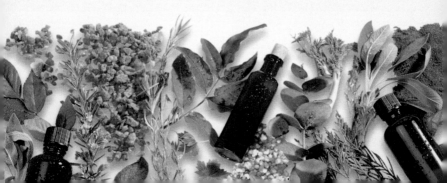

Peppermint *Mentha piperita*
Scent: Distinctive menthol-like.
Properties: Stimulant, uplifting, antiseptic, digestive, antispasmodic, pain-relieving, nerve tonic.
Uses: Indigestion, flatulence, nausea, diarrhoea, period pains, headaches, clears the mind, itchy skin conditions, bruises.
Cautions: Avoid in early pregnancy, use only well diluted on skin.

Petitgrain *Citrus aurantium*
Scent: Fresh, floral, citrus-like, woody.
Properties: Relaxant, mentally stimulating, deodorant, tonic.
Uses: Anxiety, lethargy, insomnia, stress, fear and doubts, mood uplifting, skin problems, hair tonic.
Cautions: Avoid in early pregnancy.

Rose *Rosa damascena, Rosa centifolia*
Scent: Intense rosy, floral.
Properties: Relaxant, anti-depressant, anti-spasmodic, antiseptic, sedative, nerve tonic.
Uses: Skin care, skin problems, anxiety, fears, negative emotions, menstrual problems, insomnia, headaches, nervous palpitations, depression, hangovers.
Cautions: Avoid in pregnancy.

Rosemary *Rosmarinus officinalis*
Scent: Piercing, fresh, herbaceous.
Properties: Stimulant, refreshing, tissue-warming, antiseptic, pain-relieving, antispasmodic, astringent, tonic.
Uses: Muscular stiffness and aches, arthritis, gout, headaches, neuralgia, skin problems, oily skin, water retention, respiratory problems, poor circulation, mental fatigue, poor memory.
Cautions: Avoid in pregnancy and if you have epilepsy or high blood pressure.

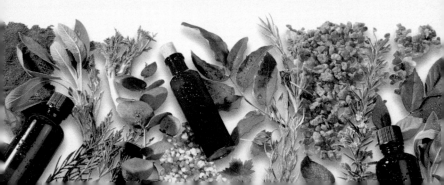

Sage, Spanish *Salvia lavandulifolia*
Scent: Camphoraceous, herby, slightly medicinal.
Properties: Stimulant, tissue-warming, antiseptic, anti-inflammatory, astringent, tonic.
Uses: Stress and tension, lethargy, mental fatigue, menstrual and menopausal problems, hormone imbalances, fluid retention, bronchial infections, colds, flu, muscular aches and joint pain, sore throat, tonsillitis, as a mild stimulant.
Cautions: Avoid in pregnancy.

Sandalwood *Santalum album*
Scent: Sweet, woody, balsamic.
Properties: Relaxant, anti-microbial, anti-depressant, antiseptic, antispasmodic, astringent, sedative, tonic, aphrodisiac.
Uses: Skin problems, throat and chest infections, stress, urinary infections, worry, fear, negative emotions.
Cautions: None.

Tea Tree *Melaleuca alternifolia*
Scent: Fresh, spicy, medicinal.
Properties: Stimulant, deodorant, anti-fungal, anti-bacterial, anti-viral, antiseptic.
Uses: Infectious conditions, cuts, sores, cold sores, herpes, ulcers, bites, skin problems, haemorrhoids, minor burns, thrush, candida, fungal vaginitis, muscular pain, athlete's foot, colds, flu, dandruff, halitosis, shock, panic, mind stimulant.
Cautions: Irritant to very sensitive skin, use well diluted for conditions like thrush, deep inhalation of neat oil can cause dizziness.

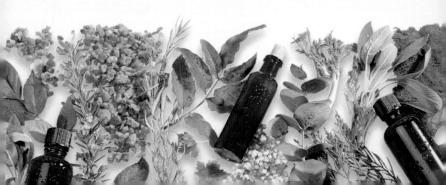

Thyme *Thymus vulgaris*
Scent: Fresh, herby.
Properties: Stimulant, anti-microbial, antiseptic.
Uses: Bronchial infections, colds, flu, sore throats, circulatory problems, rheumatic aches and pains, strengthening the immune system, mental and physical fatigue, depression, insomnia.
Cautions: Skin irritant, use well diluted, avoid in pregnancy.

Ylang Ylang *Cananga odorata*
Scent: Heavy floral, jasmine-like, smoky.
Properties: Relaxant, calming, anti-depressant, antiseptic, antifungal, deodorant, aphrodisiac, hypotensive (reducing blood pressure).
Uses: Skin care, skin problems, stress, hyperventilation, depression, anxiety, hyperactivity, stress-related high blood pressure, negative emotions.
Cautions: Avoid in early pregnancy, can cause headaches and nausea, use well diluted.

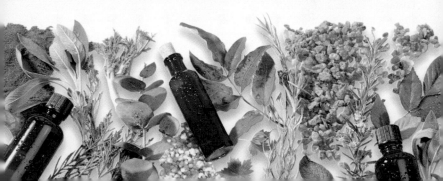

Aromatherapy
at
Home

When using essential oils it is
important to select the best
quality, and to look after them
carefully. This section gives you
advice on choosing, buying and
storing your oils, and describes
popular ways of using them.

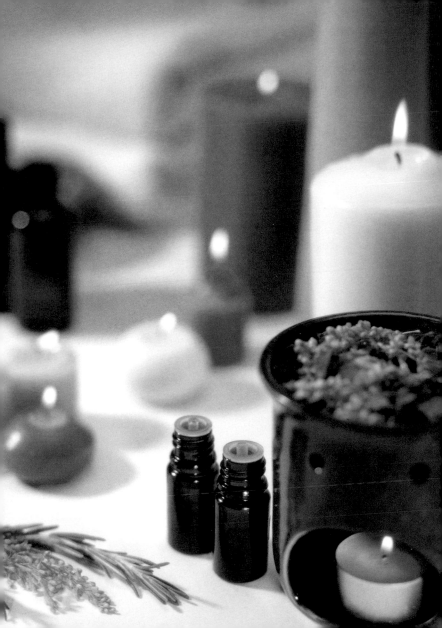

Buying essential oils

Essential oils vary enormously in price and quality. Aromatherapists say it is important the ones you select are pure essential oils, not blended. A pure oil is one that has not been adulterated with chemicals or synthetic compounds and comes from a named botanical plant from a definite geographical location. These oils will vary in price according to the yield of oil from the plant.

Some products are labelled as 'aromatherapy oils'. These are mixtures of an essential oil and a vegetable carrier oil. The proportion of essential oil in such products

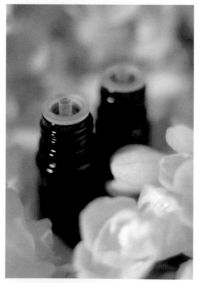

Essential oils should be stored in dark glass bottles.

varies and may be as little as 4%. A 'perfume oil' is a blend of synthetic aroma chemicals. These products are often much cheaper than pure essentials oils, but we do not know if they have a therapeutic effect.

To ensure the essential oil you buy is pure, check the label on the bottle. Responsible suppliers will also include the botanical name of the plant, and the batch code number so that the product can be traced back to its source. It is also worth smelling the oil. As a rule of thumb, if it stings your nostrils it is likely to be synthetic. Some aromatherapists suggest that for really pure essential oils, we should buy organic oils. But, with no legal controls on quality, it is difficult for consumers to establish whether oils marketed as organic are indeed so.

If you feel confused about which product to buy the best approach is to ask a qualified aromatherapist for a personal recommendation.

Storage considerations

To get the best from your essential oils you should:

- Store them in dark glass bottles in a cool dark place, as heat, light and air affect them.

- Ensure the bottle tops are tightly closed as essential oils evaporate quickly when exposed to air.

- Add the date of purchase on the bottle. Most essential oils will deteriorate after about two years, although citrus oils should be used within a year. Storing oils in the fridge can extend their effective life.

- Keep oils away from naked flames as they are flammable.

- Never store essential oils in plastic containers as this will alter the properties of the oils and may even cause the plastic to melt.

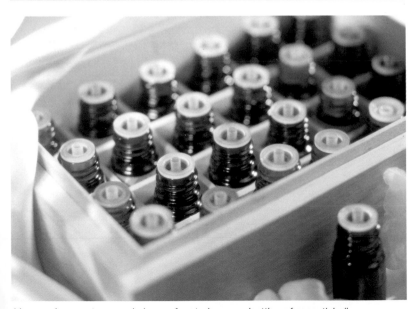

You can buy custom-made boxes for storing your bottles of essential oil.

Selecting a carrier oil

Carrier or base oils are vegetable oils that are used to dilute essential oils for use in massage or for making health and beauty preparations. Cold-pressed vegetable oils are best, because no solvents or heat have been used in the extraction process.

There are many different vegetable oils to choose from, each with different qualities. Lighter oils are good all-purpose carriers. Thick and sticky oils need to be blended with a lighter oil before use. Vegetable oils used in aromatherapy include:

- **Almond (sweet)** A light oil, suitable for most skin types, including babies. It contains vitamin E (an antioxidant that improves dry and old skin as well as helping heal burns and scars) and it keeps well.
- **Apricot kernel** A light oil, high in vitamins and minerals, and a natural moisturizer, but expensive and not easily available.
- **Avocado** A heavy oil containing vitamins A and B, lecithin, proteins and fatty acids. Readily absorbed, it is especially good for dry or older skins. Best used blended with a lighter oil.
- **Coconut** A light-textured oil suitable for all skin types. It is non-greasy, easily absorbed and nourishing.

- **Corn** A light, nourishing and inexpensive oil, suitable for all skin types.
- **Grapeseed** A light, odourless oil, easily absorbed and suitable for all skin types, especially oily skins.
- **Hazelnut** A light oil containing vitamins and minerals, easily absorbed and good for all skins, especially oily ones.
- **Jojoba** A natural liquid wax whose chemical composition resembles the skin's sebum. It contains vitamin E and has anti-bacterial properties, giving it a long shelf life. It is easily absorbed but is usually blended with lighter oils. Excellent for skin problems and facial creams.
- **Olive** A sticky oil with a strong smell, olive oil is usually used with other oils; however, it is useful for dry or sore skin.
- **Safflower** A light oil with good penetrative powers, containing minerals and vitamins. Good for all skin types and inexpensive.
- **Sesame** Extracted from raw sesame seed, this oil has a heavy

texture, contains vitamin E, and is best added to other oils.

- **Soya** A light inexpensive oil, readily absorbed and suitable for all skin types.
- **Sunflower** A light, inexpensive oil with plenty of vitamin E. Good for all skin types.
- **Wheatgerm** A dark oil with a strong smell. It is heavy and sticky but has a high vitamin E content. Added to other oils it helps guard against rancidity and prolongs the life of a blend.

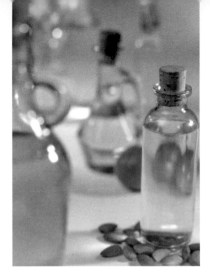

Blending guide

Blends of carrier oil and essential oils are usually divided into normal (2½%) and low (1%) dilutions, based on the amount of essential oil added.

To work out how many drops of essential oil are needed to make a normal dilution, divide the number of millilitres (ml) of carrier oil by two – for a low dilution divide by four. A full body massage requires 20ml of carrier oil. So you will need 10 drops of essential oil for a normal dilution, or five drops for a weak dilution. For babies and people with very sensitive skin use one drop of essential oil per 10ml of carrier oil; for two- to five-year-

olds use one to three drops; and for children up to the age of 12, half the quantities stated for adults.

To make a blend, choose your carrier oil and measure out the correct quantity. Decant the oil into a dark glass bottle that is a little larger than the amount of oil used. Select the essential oil or oils you require and calculate how many drops you can add. Most essential oil bottles come with a dropper for ease of measuring. Add the essential oils to the carrier. Close the top securely and label the bottle. Store in the fridge and shake well before use.

Using essential oils

Essential oils can be used in many ways. Massage is the most common, but there are a variety of ways in which you can use essential oils with beneficial effects. Here are some suggestions.

With all of the following methods, use the essential oil or oils most appropriate for the desired effect. For example, a combination of lavender and ylang ylang would be good to create a relaxing bath, and eucalyptus is excellent for clearing nasal congestion when inhaled.

- **In the bath**
  For adults, add up to six drops of essential oil(s) to a warm bath (oils will evaporate rapidly in very hot water) and agitate the water so that the oil is fully dispersed. Relax in the bath for 10–15 minutes only. People with dry skin should add the six drops of essential oil to 5ml of carrier oil first. Essential oils dissolve well in milk, so if you prefer, add your oils to a glass of milk and pour that into your bath, rather like Cleopatra!

- **Massage**
  This is the most common use of essential oils, suitably diluted in a good carrier oil. Follow the blending guidelines described earlier. Massage techniques are discussed in the next section.

- **Skin lotions and oils**
  The same principles apply here as for massage, except that the essential oils used are added to a simple cold cream or to a richer oil such as jojoba or avocado. Apply with gentle circular motions to ensure the skin is not pulled unnecessarily.

- **Neat application to the skin**
  Undiluted essential oils should not be applied to the skin, with the exception of very small amounts of lavender oil for burns, insect bites and cuts, lemon oil for warts, and tea tree oil for spots and fungal infections.

- **Hot and cold compresses**
  Compresses are a good way of using essential oils to help ease problems such as sprains, swollen joints and muscular aches. Add up to six drops of essential oil to a bowl of hot or ice-cold water. Then

dip a clean cotton cloth or a large piece of cotton wool into the solution, squeeze out the excess water and apply the compress to the affected area.

• On clothing, pillows and tissues
Add one drop of essential oil to your pillow or a tissue and inhale. Before you use an essential oil on an item of clothing, it is best to test an inconspicuous part of it with a drop of the oil.

• Steam inhalation
This is an effective way to ease nasal congestion, sinus problems and respiratory complaints. Add up to six drops of essential oil to a bowl of hot water. Inhale this under a towel.

• Vaporization
Add three to six drops of essential oil to water in a special essence burner or to a bowl of hot water to freshen a room or to create different moods.

• In room sprays
This is another way of freshening a room. Fill a plant spray with spring water and add up to 10 drops of essential oil. Shake well before use, and avoid spraying polished surfaces.

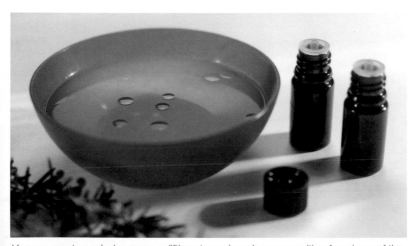

You can create a relaxing or an uplifting atmosphere in a room with a few drops of the appropriate essential oil in a bowl of hot water.

Giving a Massage

One of the most effective, not to mention pleasurable, ways of using essential oils is as part of a relaxing massage. In this section you will learn about the different massage strokes and how to give a simple massage safely.

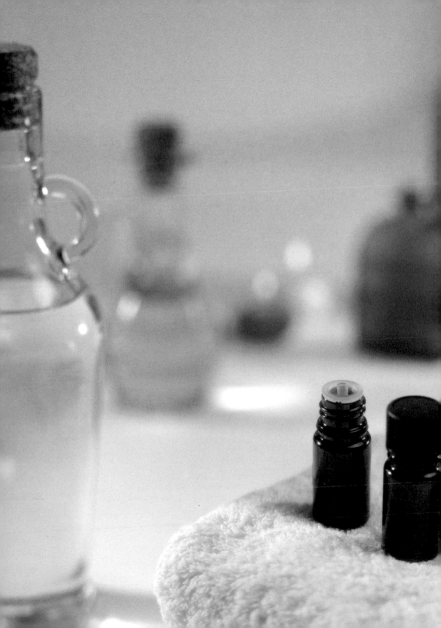

What is massage?

Massage involves the therapeutic manipulation of the soft tissues of the body (the muscles and ligaments). Massage stimulates the skin, the muscles, blood circulation and the lymphatic drainage system. It can also stimulate the release of endorphins which are the hormones that reduce the sensation of pain and increase our sense of well-being.

Soft, subdued lighting can be created by using table lamps and candles. Make sure candles are placed safely and that they are large enough to last throughout the massage.

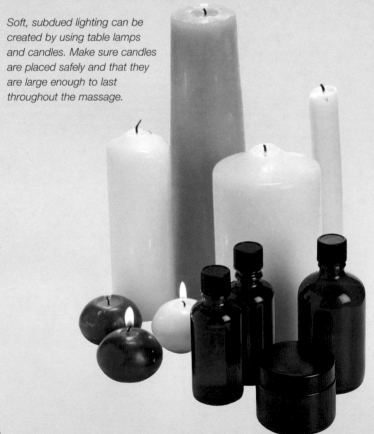

Before you start

To enhance the massage you give, choose a quiet, warm space where gentle, subdued lighting – perhaps using candles – is possible. A duvet or sleeping bag covered with towels will make an excellent surface for the person you are massaging (the receiver) to lie on. Make sure you have plenty of cushions, blankets and towels to make the receiver comfortable and to cover parts of the body not being massaged.

You should wear comfortable clothes that allow ease of movement, remove any jewellery, tie back long hair and wash your hands. Always check with the receiver before giving a massage to find out if they have any health concerns.

Select a good carrier oil in advance and ask the receiver to select the essential oil or combination of oils that feels right for them. Add up to 10 drops of essential oil to 20ml carrier oil for a full body massage.

Ask the receiver to undress – reassure them that they can leave their underwear on if they prefer. Once they are comfortable, ask them to relax and close their eyes.

When not to massage

There are certain circumstances when you should not give a massage:
- when you are feeling unwell
- if the receiver has an infectious disease, fever, acute inflammation, unexplained lumps or bumps, acute undiagnosed back pain, or has recently had surgery
- if the receiver has a serious health problem such as heart disease or thrombosis
- when the receiver is in the first three months of a pregnancy.

Make sure you have a good supply of towels and keep your essentials oils and carrier oils within easy reach.

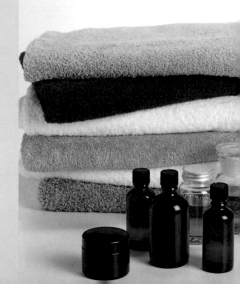

Some basic massage techniques

The most commonly used form of massage in the West is Swedish massage. This usually involves a full body massage with oils and incorporates a range of techniques which are described below.

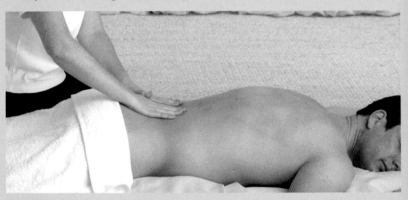

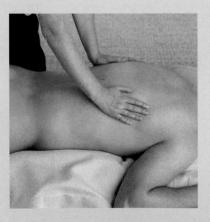

Effleurage (stroking)

This is the most basic movement. Used slowly, effluerage will relax; used briskly, it will revive and stimulate. Place your hands side by side and glide upwards, fingers leading. Then glide your hands away from each other and down the side of the area being massaged. Slowly bring your hands down the sides of the body and back to the starting position. Only apply pressure on the upward strokes.

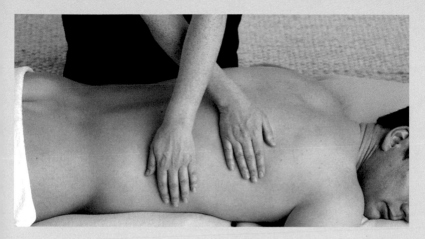

Circling

Place your hands on one side of the body and stroke round in wide curves, making a circle. As your hands meet, lift one over the other. Only exert pressure on the upward strokes.

Feathering

Brush gently over the body with your fingertips, alternating your hands. Always keep one hand on the body while taking the other hand to the starting position.

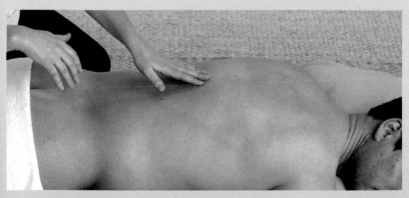

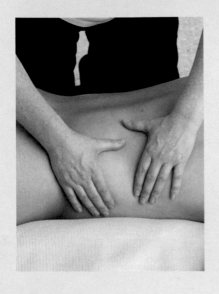

Kneading

Basic kneading involves placing both hands on the body and pressing down with the palm of one hand, grasping the flesh firmly and pushing it towards the other hand, then releasing and repeating with the other hand.

You can also exert pressure with your thumbs (place your thumbs on the body and lean your body into them) and with your knuckles (make your hand into a loose fist and apply to the body).

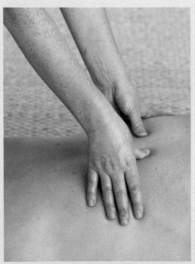

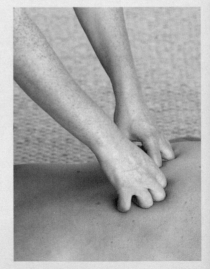

Pulling up and wringing

To 'pull up', place your hands flat on the body and grasp the muscle rather than the skin. Then pull it, firmly but gently, as far away as possible from the bone (without hurting the receiver).

Wringing is similar to wringing a towel. Start with basic kneading, then use one hand to pull the flesh up and across towards your other hand. Use the thumb of that hand to press more deeply into the flesh.

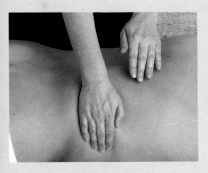

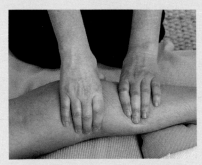

Hacking and pummelling

Lastly you can try light, brisk percussion movements such as hacking (hold your hands over the receiver with palms facing each other then flick your hands up and down

from the wrists, touching the body with the edge of your hands), and pummelling (make your hands into loose, relaxed fists and bounce the sides of your fists lightly on the skin).

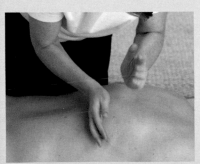

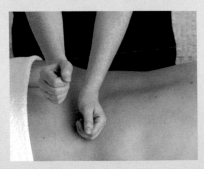

A simple body massage

To apply the oil, pour about a teaspoon into the palm of your hand, allow it to warm between your palms and then stroke it on to the receiver's body. Whatever movements you use, they should be rhythmic and the pressure used should always feel right to the receiver. Keep at least one hand on the body during the massage, and remain focused on the massage throughout. The following sequence is a very simple routine and should take about an hour.

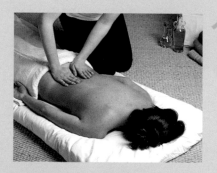

1 Start with effleurage of the back, working from the waist up to the shoulder area. Then knead up each side of the back, and use thumb pressure up each side of the spine, and pummelling, avoiding the kidneys and spine.

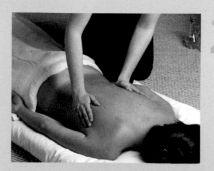

2 To finish, use some feathering strokes and then complete with light effleurage and rest your hands on the small of the back for a moment.

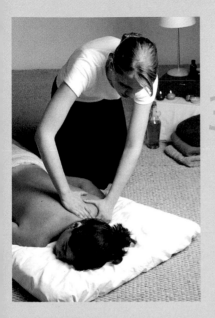

3 Next, you can work on the neck and shoulders, starting with gentle effleurage with one hand on each shoulder, working right up to the top of the neck. Then knead and use circling thumb pressure along the shoulders up to the base of the skull. Complete with light effleurage.

Before asking the receiver to turn on to their back, massage the backs of their legs using gentle effleurage. Then use firm pressure and kneading over the thigh, and pummel the outer thigh.

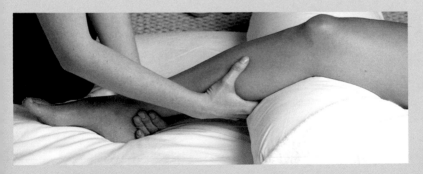

4 Next, with the receiver on their back, effleurage up from the ankles. Then raise the knee – a pillow or cushion is useful for this – and knead the calf muscles with one hand, supporting the ankle with the other. Complete with effleurage over the whole leg. Then move down to the feet.

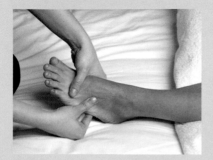

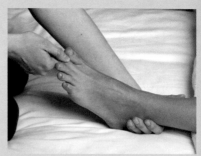

5 Use firm pressure effleurage with one hand on top of the foot, and the other underneath. Support the foot with your fingers and use thumb strokes over the top of the foot and in between the tendons.

6 Wiggle, squeeze and pull each toe and then hold them all in one hand and gently push them backwards and forwards. You can knead the soles of the foot, then finish with some gentle effleurage.

Massage the arms and hands following the same sequence.

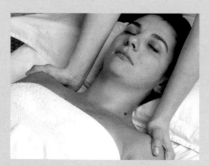

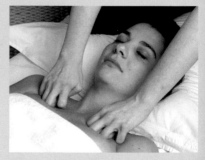

7 Next, massage the chest and neck. First kneel behind the head and place a hand on each shoulder, fingers facing towards the floor. Lean into the shoulders to stretch and loosen the muscles.

8 Then use kneading, thumb pressure and knuckling over the whole area.

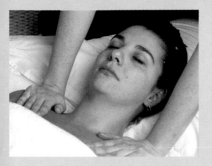

9 Finish with gentle effleurage.

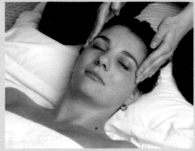

10 To massage the face you might want to use an enriched face cream containing essential oils, or a special face oil. To spread the oil or cream, place both hands on the neck and use effleurage over the neck, up the chin and side of the face to the ears. Then glide back down to the neck.

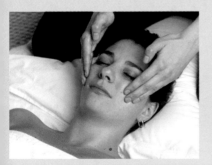

11 Stroke the neck, chin, mouth and round the nostrils using your finger tips. Work across the cheekbones to the temples and back down to the chin.

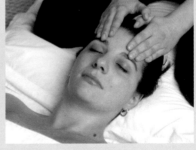

12 Place your hands across the forehead, fingers touching, and stroke outwards using your fingers. Also use circular pressure over the forehead. Finish by placing both hands over the face for a minute.

Aromatherapy *for* Health *Problems*

Aromatherapy can help enhance our health and sense of well-being. It can also be used to treat minor health problems. This section will suggest safe aromatherapy treatments for a range of common ailments.

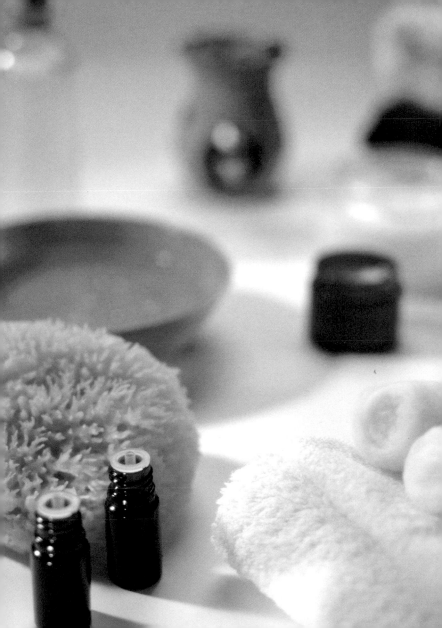

Some simple rules

It is important to use this section in conjunction with all the previous sections, and to follow the blending guidelines given throughout.

We know that most health problems can have more than one cause. Similarly, there is usually more than one helpful essential oil. You will need to experiment to find the oil or combination of oils which works for you. Just smelling the suggested oils will guide you – simply avoid the aromas you do not like!

The remedies given here are for adults, not children. For beginners, it is probably safest to stick to treating adults and to avoid using essential oils in pregnancy. Aromatherapy can be very helpful, but it requires considerable experience to use essential oils appropriately for pregnant women or small children.

While these remedies have been used successfully by many people, if there is no improvement within a day or two, you should seek medical advice.

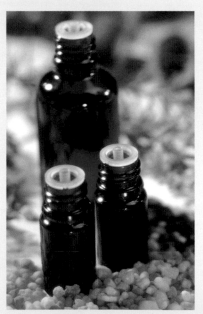

When preparing your treatment oils, remember to stick to the following blending guidelines:

Massage: *20ml carrier oil to 10 drops essential oil (normal dilution)*
Bath: *Up to six drops essential oil*
Compress (hot or cold): *Up to six drops essential oil*
Steam inhalation: *Up to six drops essential oil in a bowl of hot water*
Neat: *one to two drops essential oil*
Essence burner: *six drops essential oil*

An A–Z of common health problems

ACHES AND PAINS
Backache
Oils: Lavender, lemon, melissa, orange, Roman camomile, rosemary
Treatments:
- Soothing back massage.
- A therapeutic bath.

Cramp
Oils: Clary sage, cypress, lavender marjoram
Treatments:
- Rub affected area with massage blend.
- After an attack of cramp, a bath with a mixture of lavender, marjoram and camomile will help relax muscles.

Headaches
Oils: Eucalyptus, geranium, lavender, lemon, marjoram, peppermint, rose, rosemary
Treatments:
- Use an essence burner.
- A therapeutic bath.
- Shoulder, neck, face and scalp massage with circular pressure.
- Rub a drop of neat lavender oil into temples.

Muscular aches and pains
Oils: Eucalyptus, blue camomile, lavender, marjoram, rosemary
Treatments:
- Gentle massage over affected area.
- A therapeutic bath.

DIGESTIVE PROBLEMS
Constipation
Oils: Lemongrass, marjoram, orange, rosemary
Treatments:
- Massage abdomen and around navel, finish with foot massage.
- A therapeutic bath.

Diarrhoea
Oils: Lemon, neroli, peppermint, Roman camomile, sandalwood
Treatments:
- Very gentle massage over abdomen, with carrier oil containing equal parts of the above oils, or equal parts peppermint and camomile (or sandalwood).
- Warm compress to abdomen with same combinations of essential oils.

Indigestion
Oils: Fennel, lavender, orange, peppermint, Roman camomile, rosemary
Treatments:
- Gentle massage clockwise around abdomen.

- Put one drop of peppermint oil on a handkerchief and inhale.

Nausea
Oils: Lavender, orange, peppermint, petitgrain
Treatments:
- Put two drops of essential oil on a handkerchief and inhale.
- Add peppermint oil to an essence burner.

INFECTIONS AND RESPIRATORY PROBLEMS
Catarrh and sinusitis
Oils: Cypress, eucalyptus, fennel, frankincense, lavender, marjoram, myrrh, peppermint, rosemary, sandalwood, tea tree
Treatments:
- Massage with gentle circular pressure around base of the skull, eyebrows, forehead and base of nose. Finish with light stroking over whole area.
- Steam inhalation.
- Place two drops of essential oil on a handkerchief and inhale.
- Use an essence burner.

Chest infections (bronchitis, etc.)
Oils: Bergamot, cypress, eucalyptus, frankincense, lavender, marjoram, peppermint, sandalwood, Spanish sage, tea tree

Treatments:
- Chest massage.
- Steam inhalation.
- A therapeutic bath.

Colds , coughs and flu
Oils: Bergamot, cypress, eucalyptus, frankincense, lavender, lemon, marjoram, rosemary, tea tree, thyme
Treatments:
- Chest, neck and face massage.
- Steam inhalation.
- A therapeutic bath – good combinations are equal parts lavender, bergamot and tea tree; or equal parts lavender, thyme and tea tree.
- Use equal parts lavender, lemon and tea tree in an essence burner.

Sore throat
Oils: Bergamot, clary sage, cypress, geranium, lavender, lemon, peppermint, sandalwood, tea tree
Treatments:
- Gentle stroking massage to the throat area.
- Gargle with a cup of warm water with one teaspoon honey and two drops each of lavender, lemon and tea tree. Do not swallow.
- Warm compress to affected area.

THE MIND AND EMOTIONS
Anxiety
Oils: Bergamot, clary sage, frankincense, lavender, lemon, patchouli, petitgrain, Roman camomile, rose, sandalwood, thyme
Treatments:
- Gentle massage to solar plexus to relieve tightness in the stomach.
- A therapeutic bath – for the morning try equal parts bergamot and frankincense, and for the evening, equal parts sandalwood, ylang ylang and thyme.
- Use same combinations of oils in an essence burner.
- Face lotion – 10ml base, four drops each of rose and sandalwood, or four drops each of petitgrain and clary sage. Use as required.

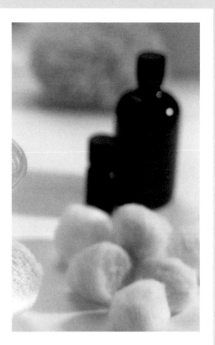

Grief
Oils: Cypress, jasmine, lavender, marjoram, Roman camomile, rose
Treatments:
- Sniff the bottles as for smelling salts for shock.
- Use an essence burner.
- Add two drops to your pillow at night.
- Regular therapeutic baths.
- Face oil – 10ml base, eight drops rose or jasmine, or four drops of each. Use daily initially then once or twice a week as required.

Mild depression
Oils: Bergamot, clary sage, frankincense, geranium, jasmine, lavender, melissa, neroli, orange, patchouli, Roman camomile, rose, Spanish sage, sandalwood, ylang ylang
Treatments:
- Full body massage.
- Therapeutic baths.
- Use an essence burner – a good combination is equal parts sweet basil, bergamot, melissa, sandalwood and ylang ylang.

• Face oil – 20ml base oil and five drops each of neroli, orange and petitgrain. Use regularly.

Poor memory
Oils: Rosemary, sweet basil, thyme
Treatment:
• Use an essence burner regularly.

SKIN AND HAIR PROBLEMS
Acne
Oils: Bergamot, blue camomile, geranium, lavender, lemon, lemongrass, petitgrain, Roman camomile, sandalwood, tea tree
Treatments:
• Regular gentle face massage.
• If very inflamed, apply a cold compress.
• Use a gentle skin tonic to cleanse skin. A good formula is 10ml vodka, 100ml distilled water, 10 drops each of Blue camomile and petitgrain and four drops tea tree.
• Use diluted tea tree on spots using a cotton wool bud.

Dandruff
Oils: Cypress, lavender, rosemary
Treatment:
• Add three drops essential oil to 10ml jojoba oil and massage into scalp. Shampoo with unscented shampoo (you can add five drops of essential oil to 10ml shampoo if you wish). After shampooing, rinse normally, but apply a final rinse mix of 10ml water, 5ml vinegar and three drops rosemary.

Eczema
Oils: Bergamot, blue camomile, frankincense, geranium, lavender, patchouli, rose, sandalwood, tea tree, ylang ylang
Treatments:
• Gentle full body massage – use well diluted and always do a patch test first. For dry eczema try a mix of bergamot, geranium and sandalwood, lavender or tea tree. For weeping eczema try a mix of patchouli and cedarwood or rose.
• For dry eczema try therapeutic baths, diluting the essential oils before adding.

Stress
Oils: Frankincense, lavender, lemongrass, marjoram, neroli, orange, petitgrain, Roman camomile, sandalwood
Treatments:
• A regular full body massage.
• Regular therapeutic baths – good combinations include equal parts lavender and frankincense, or lavender and marjoram.
• Use an essence burner.

STRESS-RELATED PROBLEMS
Insomnia
Oils: Bergamot, clary sage, frankincense, lavender, marjoram, neroli, orange, petitgrain, Roman camomile
Treatments:
- Use an essence burner in the evening.
- Before bed try a relaxing bath – good combinations include equal parts lavender and bergamot, neroli and camomile, or camomile and lavender.
- Put two drops of lavender or ylang ylang on your pillow.

Mental fatigue or nervous exhaustion
Oils: Clary sage, lemongrass, peppermint, rosemary
Treatments:
- Gentle face massage and scalp massage.
- Use peppermint oil in an essence burner.
- Steam inhalation.

Lack of confidence
Oils: Bergamot, clary sage, frankincense, geranium, jasmine, orange, Roman camomile, rose, sandalwood
Treatments:
- A regular full body massage.
- Regular therapeutic baths.

Depression and lethargy
Oils: Bergamot, clary sage, geranium, jasmine, lavender, melissa, orange and sandalwood
Treatments:
- Full body massage, plus an invigorating foot massage or scalp massage.
- A therapeutic bath.

WOMEN'S HEALTH PROBLEMS
Menstrual problems – PMT and period pains
Oils: Clary sage, cypress, geranium, jasmine, lavender, marjoram, melissa, peppermint, Roman camomile, rose
Treatments:
- Gentle back and abdomen massage.
- A therapeutic bath.
- Apply warm compress to abdomen.

Menopause – Hot flushes
Oils: Cypress, Spanish sage
Treatment:
- Massage feet each night before going to bed.

Menopause – Mood swings
Oils: Geranium, clary sage, lavender, petitgrain
Treatments:
- Use an essence burner.
- Regular therapeutic baths.

First Aid

We all have a medicine cupboard ready for those everyday emergencies and problems. Here are some suggestions of where aromatherapy can also help.

Athlete's foot

Oils: Clary sage, geranium, lemongrass, tea tree
Treatments:

• Mix 10ml soya oil and two drops each of wheatgerm oil, tea tree and geranium. Rub between toes and around nails daily. You can substitute almond for soya oil, and lemongrass for tea tree and geranium.
• Bathe feet in a bowl of salted water containing five drops of tea tree or clary sage. Soak for at least 10 minutes, then dry thoroughly.

Bruises

Oils: Lavender, tea tree
Treatment:

• Cold compresses.

Chilblains

Oil: Tea tree
Treatments:

• Apply one drop of neat tea tree to the affected area.
• Massage feet with 10ml grapeseed oil and five drops tea tree.

Cold sores

Oils: Lavender, tea tree
Treatment:

• Dilute essential oil in carrier oil and dab on cold sore with a cotton wool bud.

Earache

Oils: Lavender, Roman camomile, tea tree
Treatment:

• Massage around ear and jaw, including gentle circular pressure.

Insect bites and stings

Oils: Blue or Roman camomile, lavender, tea tree
Treatments:

• Apply one drop of neat lavender or tea tree to the affected area (pull sting out with tweezers if visible).
• Apply a cold compress with two drops each of lavender and camomile to areas of swelling.

Jetlag

Oils: Calming – Geranium, lavender, clary sage. Uplifting – Bergamot, peppermint, rosemary
Treatments:

• To promote sleep, inhale two drops of a calming oil on a handkerchief, and/or try a gentle shoulder massage or foot massage.

- To revive yourself, inhale two drops of an uplifting oil on a handkerchief, add up to six drops of essential oils to a bath, or give yourself an energetic foot massage.

Minor burns
Oils: Lavender, tea tree, Roman camomile
Treatment:
- Immerse the burn in cold water till the pain subsides, then apply a small amount of neat lavender or tea tree to the affected area, or use a cold compress with two drops each of lavender and camomile.

Minor cuts and grazes
Oils: Blue camomile, lavender, tea tree
Treatments:
- Wash with cool water, then apply a cold compress.
- Apply a drop of neat lavender to the cleaned wound to help with healing, and cover with a plaster, if necessary.

Mouth ulcers
Oils: Myrrh, tea tree, thyme
Treatments:
- Apply one drop neat tea tree using a cotton bud – blot area with tissue to remove excess oil before closing mouth or swallowing.

- Rinse mouth with a mouthwash made of two drops myrrh and two drops thyme in a glass of warm water. Do not swallow. Use twice a day.

Panic attacks
Oils: Clary sage, frankincense, lavender, rose, sweet basil, tea tree
Treatments:
- Waft a bottle of frankincense, lavender or tea tree under the nose like smelling salts, but avoid inhaling too deeply.
- Massage solar plexus area.

Sprains and strains
Oils: Blue or Roman camomile, cypress, frankincense, lavender, marjoram, rosemary
Treatment:
- Elevate affected area if possible and use a cold compress.

Sunburn
Oils: Bergamot, lavender, sandalwood, Roman camomile
Treatments:
- Apply a few drops of neat lavender to affected areas to ease the pain.
- Apply after-sun lotion made of 50ml base, six drops bergamot, six drops lavender, five drops camomile, and five drops sandalwood to affected areas.

Making
Aromatherapy
Toiletries

The shelves of health food shops, chemists and supermarkets are laden with 'aromatherapy' products. From bath oils to skin toners, and foot spas to aftershaves, their wonderful aromas and attractive packaging entice even the most hardened of shoppers. Yet it is actually very easy to make your own aromatherapy toiletries and the end product will be well worth the effort!

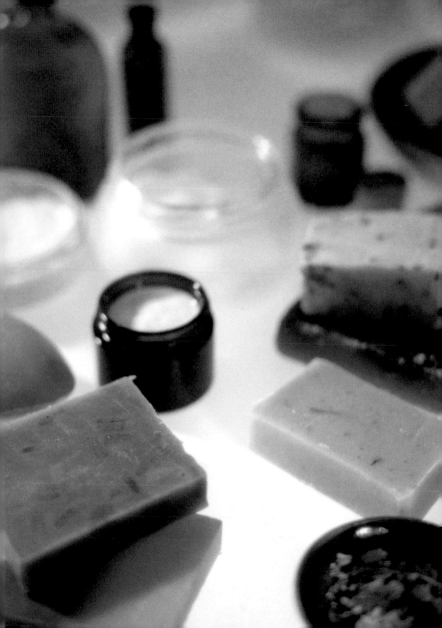

Getting started

Before embarking on any of the recipes in this section, it is important to review the information regarding safety guidelines, and buying and storing essential oils. You should also follow the blending directions given and not be tempted to use more of any essential oil mentioned. That said, the most important thing to do is to have fun!

Bath products

Apart from the obvious need to get clean or just having a relaxing soak, having a bath can be beneficial for your health and sense of well-being. Using essential oils will, at the very least, add a great 'feel-good factor' to your cleansing routine. You can either make up a bath oil as and when you want one, or make up a larger quantity and store it. The therapeutic qualities of the bath oils you make will last up to three months if stored correctly.

The recipes given here are the quantities you will need for one full bath. Mix the oils together first and then add to a filled bath. If you want to soften your skin and remove impurities, dissolve two cups of Epsom salts in the bath water before adding your bath oil. You should get in the bath immediately after adding the mixture as the essential oils evaporate quite quickly. Then, simply relax and enjoy your bath for up to half an hour.

Muscle-relaxing bath oil
3 drops cypress oil
2 drops marjoram oil
2 drops lavender oil
1 drop sweet basil oil
1 drop cedarwood oil
5ml carrier oil (e.g. sweet almond, grapeseed or hazelnut)

Uplifting bath oil
3 drops geranium oil
2 drops bergamot oil
1 drop allspice oil
1 drop orange oil
5ml carrier oil

Refreshing bath oil
3 drops rosemary oil
3 drops bergamot oil
5ml carrier oil

Calming bath oil
2 drops petitgrain oil
2 drops ylang ylang oil
2 drops orange oil
5ml carrier oil

Hair care

We all aspire to soft, shiny hair and these aromatherapy conditioners will help you achieve just that. Massage 5ml of the conditioner into your hair and scalp. Wrap a towel round your head and keep it there for a few hours, to allow the oils to penetrate. Then wash your hair twice with a natural shampoo (available from health food shops and pharmacies), using warm, not hot, water. For best results use the conditioner three times a week until you are happy with the results, then use occasionally as required. These mixtures will keep for around three months.

Conditioner for normal hair
8 drops thyme oil
6 drops sage oil
6 drops Roman camomile oil
5 drops lavender oil
30ml jojoba carrier oil

Conditioner for oily hair
8 drops petitgrain oil
8 drops lemon oil
8 drops lavender oil
30ml hazelnut carrier oil

Conditioner for dry hair
10 drops sandalwood oil
10 drops bois de rose oil
5 drops palmarosa oil
30ml jojoba carrier oil

Footbath

After a long walk or a hard day at work, a relaxing foot bath will do wonders for your sense of well-being. The quantities given below are enough for one footbath, but, as with other recipes, you can always make more and store it in a clean, dry bottle with a well-fitting lid. Add the mixture to a washing-up bowl and disperse the blended oils. Relax with your feet in the water for at least 15 minutes.

Relaxing foot bath
3 drops myrrh oil
3 drops Roman camomile oil
3 drops orange oil
2 drops lemon oil
5ml carrier oil

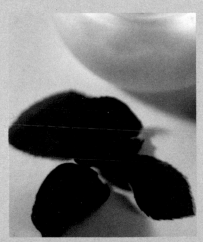

Skin care

This preparation can be used as a cleansing cream, a moisturizing cream or as an alternative to oil in certain sorts of massage. The cream can be kept in small individual jars, and different essential oils added to each depending on your requirements. Each batch will last several weeks as the essential oils seem to act as natural preservatives.

Simple skin cream
20g almond carrier oil
10g shredded beeswax (use a sharp knife for shredding)
40g rosewater, orange-flower water or distilled water
10 drops essential oil

Add the almond oil and beeswax to a Pyrex bowl and place in a shallow pan of water over a gentle heat. Stir until the ingredients have melted, then turn off the heat.

Add the rosewater to the oil mixture, a drop or two at a time, while beating the mixture with a whisk (you can use an electric whisk if you wish). When all the rosewater has been absorbed, divide the mixture into small jars.

Add the essential oil required to these jars. Essential oils which are suitable even for sensitive skin include jasmine, rose, geranium, lavender and neroli.

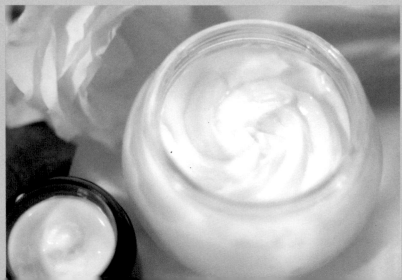

Skin preparations

To help rejuvenate your skin, wash thoroughly first, then massage one of these preparations into your skin. This can be repeated daily. The ingredients should be mixed together by shaking in a clean, dry bottle with a cap.

• for normal skin
10 drops lavender oil
10 drops palmarosa oil
10 drops geranium oil
30ml hazelnut carrier oil

• for dry skin
10 drops sandalwood oil
10 drops bois de rose oil
10 drop lavender oil
30ml avocado carrier oil

• for oily skin
10 drops ylang ylang oil
10 drops lemon oil
5 drops cypress oil
5 drops petitgrain oil
30ml grapeseed carrier oil

Toners

Skin toning is an important part of any cleansing routine. The following are sweet-smelling aromatherapy alternatives to the many commercial products on the market. Keep them in a sealed, clean, dry bottle and shake well before use.

• for sensitive skin
4 drops blue camomile
10ml vodka
250ml distilled water

• for oily skin
3 drops bergamot oil
3 drops lavender oil
15ml vodka
250ml orange-flower water
  (available from pharmacies, health food shops and supermarkets)

• for normal skin
3 drops palmarosa oil
3 drops rose oil
15ml vodka
250ml rosewater (available from pharmacies, health food shops and supermarkets)

• for dry skin
4 drops rose absolute oil
2 drops Roman camomile oil
20ml vodka

Aftershave

For a gentle aftershave for sensitive skin, or for teenagers embarking on shaving for the first time, add the following to a clean, dry bottle with a well-fitting cap and shake well:

25ml vodka
250ml orange-flower water
  (available from good pharmacies)
6 drops essential oil

After making this mixture, you can add an oil to give it an aroma. As this is such a personal choice, it's best to leave it to the recipient. However, a good choice is sandalwood as it is said to have anti-bacterial properties, and those who use it in aftershaves do say it is very helpful with the rashes that can be an inevitable result of shaving. Always give the bottle a good shake before using the aftershave.

Mouthwash

This recipe to help freshen your mouth and breath will make a concentrated mouthwash which can then be added to water as required. The usual proportions are 2–3 teaspoons of mouthwash to half a glass (of average size) of warm water. Some people prefer to add the concentrate to pure bottled water. To make the mouthwash, add the following ingredients to a clean, dry bottle with a secure cap and shake well:

125ml cheap brandy
15 drops thyme oil
15 drops peppermint oil
5 drops myrrh oil
5 drops fennel oil

Always shake the bottle well before using the mouthwash.

Useful contacts

The following organizations will supply you with further information:

Aromatherapy and Allied Practitioners' Association
8 George Street, Croydon, Surrey
CR0 1PA
Tel: +44 (0)20 8680 7761
www.aromatherapyuk@aol.com
www.aapa.org.uk

Aromatherapy Organizations Council (AOC)
PO Box 19834, London SE25 6WF
Tel: +44 (0)20 8251 7912
Fax: +44 (0)20 8251 7942
www.aromatherapy-uk.org
Umbrella group representing the main professional aromatherapy associations

Association of Medical Aromatherapists
11 Park Circus, Glasgow G3 6AX
Tel: 0141 3324924
Compuserv.com/homepage/
complementarymedicinecentre

International Federation of Aromatherapists (IFA)
182 Chiswick High Road, London
W4 1PP
Tel: +44 (0)20 8742 2605
www.int-fedaromatherapy.co.uk

International Society of Professional Aromatherapists
82 Ashby Road, Hinkley,
Leicestershire LE10 1SN
Tel: +44 (01)455 637987
e-mail: admin@the-ifpa.org
www.the-ispa.org
The largest group in the AOC

American Institute of Massage Therapy, Inc
2101 North, Federal Highway, Fort
Lauderdale, Florida 33305
Tel: +1 954 568 6200
Fax: +1 954 568 6100

Australian Natural Therapists Association
PO Box 522, Sutherland, NSW 2232
Tel: +61 (02) 521 2063

Canadian Massage Therapist Alliance
365 Bloor Street East, Suite 1807,
Toronto, Ontario M4W 3L4
Tel: +1 416 968 2149
Fax: +1 416 968 6818

N.B. If dialling from outside the country, use the appropriate international dialling codes.

Index